I HAVE A FRIEND
IN A WHEELCHAIR

HANNAH CARLSON, M.ED, CRC
DALE CARLSON

illustrated by
HOPE M. DOUGLAS, M.A.

CHANEY SHANNON PRESS
BICK PUBLISHING HOUSE
MADISON, CT

Text © copyright 1995 by Hannah Carlson, M.ED., CRC
and Dale Carlson
© illustrations 1995 by Hope M. Douglas, M. A.
© cover and book design 1995 by Jane Miller Productions

Edited by Ann Maurer

With thanks to Richard Fucci, former president
National Spinal Cord Injury Association

CHANEY SHANNON PRESS is a trademark of
BICK PUBLISHING HOUSE

Library of Congress Catalog Card Number: 95-79843

ISBN: 1-884158-09-9—Volume 4
ISBN: 1-884158-11-0—4 Volume Set

Printed by Royal Printing Service, Guilford, CT, USA

Special needs/disabilities

"These books are an important service. They are informed, practical guides to feelings, behavior patterns, medical facts, technology, and resources for people who care about people with disabilities."
    –Richard Fucci, former president of the National Spinal
      Cord Injury Association

"Excellent, very informative."
    –Alan R. Ecker, M.D., Assistant Clinical Professor of
      Opthalmology, Yale University

"An invaluable source of help and comfort for friends and caregivers of people who have disabilities or special needs."
    –Mary Jon Edwards, Nationally Certified Therapeutic
      Horseback Riding Instructor, Special Olympics

"Excellent introductory handbooks about disabilities and special needs. They discuss medical conditions and rehabilitation, feelings and adaptive technology, and responsible attitudes both on the part of people with disabilities and people temporarily without them. The emphasis is on our common humanity, not our differences."
    –Lynn McCrystal, M.ED.,vice-president, The Kennedy Center

"The books offer professional information in an easy-to-use, uncomplicated style."
    –Renee Abbott, Group Home Director, S.A.R.A.H.,
      Shoreline Association for the Retarded and Handicapped

"Precise information, good reading for the layperson."
    –Jane Chamberlin, parent and employment supervisor, West
      Haven Community House

"Thank you for the opportunity to be a part of this work."
    –Christine M. Gaglio, employment specialist for the deaf, The
      Kennedy Center

CONTENTS

NOTE

It is hard to be different, to feel alone, to be rendered power-less. Millions of people in the United States live with what are said to be disabilities. If you are family, caregiver, old friend or new friend, recognize that it is hard to sit in a wheelchair in a world so insistent on standing tall, that equates self-worth with independence, and regards any handicap as a failure. The lives of many people with disabilities have not significantly improved, even with the passage of the Americans with Disabilities Act and the federal deinstitutionalization policy. Too often a person with a disability undergoes a kind of social death long before experiencing a physical one.

Understanding the needs and feelings of anyone is a require-ment for friendship, for relationship. This is just as true for a person in a wheelchair or on crutches. Understanding can also relieve us of the misinformation that to be in a wheelchair is nec-essarily to be in any more distress than anyone else. There are resources for information, help, and reassurance to remind us that we are all in this together.

ACKNOWLEDGMENTS

Our gratitude to Theodore Harold Bromm and Renee Abbott, Group Home Director, both of S.A.R.A.H., the Shoreline Association of the Retarded and Handicapped; to Richard Fucci, former president of the National Spinal Cord Injury Association; to Alan Ecker, M.D. Assistant Clinical Professor of Opthalmology, Yale; to Jane Chamberlin, parent and employment supervisor, West Haven Community House; and to Lynn McCrystal, M.Ed., vice-president, The Kennedy Center, for their counsel and editorial advice.

Our gratitude to Louis and Susan Weady, not only for Royal Printing, but for their guidance and patience with new editions, purchase orders, and shipping.

Our special thanks to Herb Swartz for his kindness and the use of his computers.

Our further special thanks to Danny Carlson for teaching us how to use computer capabilities for publishing.

And our thanks to Terrence Finnegan for providing Bick Publishing House with its own computer system.

1

WHEELCHAIRS AND CRUTCHES: CAUSES AND CONDITIONS

There are a lot of reasons people are in wheelchairs. Some conditions began before or during birth. Some conditions were acquired. Some are painful, some are a physical nuisance.

They include:

Trauma

Genetic disorders, birth defects and injury

Chronic, acute, and terminal diseases

Weakening and loss of physical abilities in the elderly

TRAUMA

Trauma is the most common cause of death in young people; head injury, followed by spinal cord injury, accounts for half of these trauma-related deaths. Car and motorcycle crashes, war, crime (especially gunshot wounds), and sports injuries, the accident of being in the wrong place at the wrong time are major arenas for injury.

These accidents can result in the need for adaptive equipment. Some conditions may result in the need for a wheelchair, or for arm, leg, or neck braces, for crutches or for canes.

Amputation of one or both legs

TBI (traumatic brain injury)

Spinal cord injury

TBI or spinal cord injury may result in limb weakness or paralysis. TBI may cause hemiplegia (paralysis on one side). Paraplegia (paralysis of legs)or quadriplegia (paralysis of arms and legs), possibly even the respiratory system, will depend on the level of injury to the spinal cord, itself nerve tissue, from which issue all nerves to the trunk and limb. The higher the level of injury to the spinal cord, the more nerves are paralyzed.

GENETIC DISORDERS, BIRTH DEFECTS AND INJURY
Genetic Disorders

Chromosomes are the vehicles in which the genes are carried from generation to generation. Virtually all characteristics, and this includes diseases as well as human traits such as personality, height, and intelligence, are to some extent determined by the genes.

Genetic changes, alterations, disorders, are termed mutations. These can be inherited or spontaneous, and can produce congenital anomalies.

Absence of lower limbs.

Spina bifida: congenital defect in walls of spinal canal, vertebrae or cord abnormalities

Abnormalities of lower limb bones, muscles, and nervous system that result in weakness, wasting, deformity, contracture.

Birth Defects and Injury

Genetic disorders are often referred to as birth defects, but there is also a group of conditions arising either from the birth process itself, or the mother's health and condition during pregnancy.

Strangling umbilical cord: if the brain is deprived of oxygen for too long, there may be paralysis or developmental defects

Drugs: the mother's ingestion of alcohol, cocaine, or other improper drugs, can affect proper development of the fetus. As an example, the drug thalidomide, once prescribed for pregnant women, caused babies to be born with deformed or absent limbs

Improper nutrition and prenatal care

Conditions in the mother's health, such as HIV or AIDS, can produce lifelong disabilities in the child

ACUTE, CHRONIC, AND TERMINAL DISEASES

Many diseases affect the ability to control muscles well enough to walk.

Myasthenia gravis is a neuromuscular disorder that weakens many muscle groups of the face and head as well as the limbs. Nerve impulses fail to induce normal muscle contractions. Activity only increases the weakness.

Cerebral palsy, of either the limp or spastic kind, is the loss of ability to move or to control movement. It may be mild, or severe enough to require life in a wheelchair. It is not progressive, but it cannot be reversed. It results from developmental defects in the brain or trauma at birth.

Other palsies can be either genetic or acquired. Some are progressive like Parkinson's, some nonprogressive like those caused by birth trauma.

Leprosy, AIDS, polio, Lyme are infectious and inflammatory diseases that can produce associated neuropathies, that is, diseases of the nerves.

Acquired disabilities such as heart, vascular, and artery diseases can cause stroke and aneurysm that result in paralysis. There are tumors, both benign and cancerous, that can cause either paralysis or general weakness. Cancer and diabetes are among the diseases that can result in amputations that necessitate wheelchairs or crutches.

ICI means invisible, chronic illness. ICI's do not necessarily have visible symptoms. Often the causes are unknown, but all are characterized by alternating periods of exacerbation (a flare-up of symptoms) and remission (lessening of symptoms), and can so weaken the body that wheelchair or crutches may be necessary. ICI's include multiple sclerosis, a progressive disease of the central nervous system, IBS (irritable bowel syndrome), endometriosis, lupus, chronic fatigue immunodeficiency syndrome. There are others. ICI's are not terminal, but cause a lifetime of pain, fatigue, and incapacity to the person afflicted.

Age is a condition that sometimes requires the use of wheelchair or crutches, canes or walkers. While the mind can stay young and fresh, biology marches on, and bodies can get old and infirm and require a bit of mobility assistance.

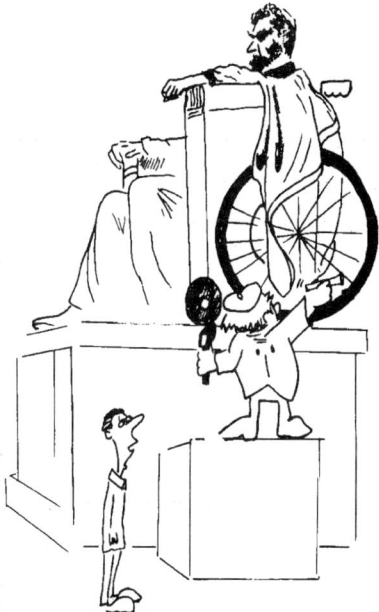

Please. Don't you think he's special enough?

2

THEIR FEELINGS, YOUR FEELINGS

Disability can be a redemption from the ordinary thoughtless busyness that makes most people race to the finish, look back at their lives, and ask, "What was that?"

Disability can be an invitation to self-examination and meditation, and, because it slows you down, an invitation to awareness. The authors share a disability, and it has turned our lives into more deeply felt experience.

Disability can also be an invitation to ingenuity.

• Ed Roberts, quadriplegic at 14, unable to move below the neck execpt for a finger, dependent on an iron lung to breathe, said it was the paternalism of others, more than his own disability, that held him back, and with his portable respirator at his back, talked his way into the University of California, and inspired other rolling quads to enroll. They put ramps on campus housing, set up a 24-hour emergency wheelchair repair service, and hired attendants to help with personal care. Today, there are 300 independent living centers on the Berkeley model across America. Some of the first sidewalk curb cuts were built for him. As president of the World Institute on Disability, he taught the 49 million people with disabilities that attitudes were a bigger problem than their disabilities.

• Marilyn Hamilton, athlete, crashed into a mountain while she was handgliding. She never walked again. But she played tennis, skiied, and used her need for swift, lightweight motion to advance the invention of mobile, lightweight wheelchairs so that her movements were liberated, not bound, by her wheelchair.

• Ed Tessier, quadriplegic and political candidate for Congress, was not going to wait for the research of the Miami Project to discover how to repair the nerves of the spinal cord for the nearly 2 million people in wheelchairs. Nor was he interested in the FES(functional electrical stimulus) parastep walkers at $15,000 each to get him on his feet. He feels the medical model is a trap. He prefers not to postpone his life and wait for cures, but to be the first quad in Congress and campaign against the segregation of stairs and narrow doors and entrances through the kitchen for his own minority, as well as to fight prejudice for all minorities.

Remarkable Rehabilitants

John Callahan, cartoonist
Franklin Roosevelt, President of the United States
Kathy Martin and Ben Hogen, athletes
Milton Erikson, psychiatrist
Stephen Hawking, physicist and cosmologist

THEIR FEELINGS

There is always the dark side. The disabled experience an

agony of self-hate, the fear of being helpless, worthless, unloved and unloving. And different, relentlessly, permanently, different.

Most illnesses follow a path from warning signs to recovery or death. Visible disabilities or invisible chronic illnesses are characterized by the worst fears that plague us all: unmitigated pain; the helpless dependency; death.

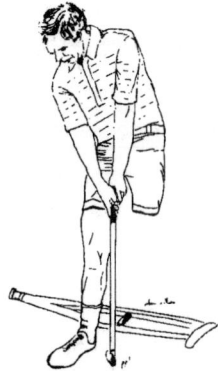

Dick Heartwell
Amputee, Handicap 7

There may be continuous discomfort, feelings of insecurity in relationships, the anxiety and despair of loneliness, often deep depression, sometimes shame, and the sad feeling of being left out of life's party. The daily management of pain, and planning the simple, difficult details of daily living in a wheelchair or on crutches can require so much energy that someone with a disability might easily lose the ability to focus attention on the broad goals of a well-lived life.

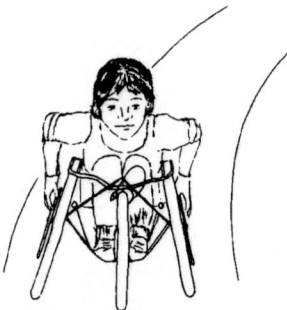

Kathy Martin, Marathon racer

Some other possible feelings:

guilt: am I bad, or irresponsible? is this a punishment? is it my fault? am I too much of a burden on others?

anger: at the self for having the disability, at oth-

13

ers for not; at another for causing it; at society for treating those who have it as pariahs ·

low self-esteem: among those with TBI and spinal cord injury, as well as in severe cerebral palsy, some ICI's such as multiple sclerosis, sexual dysfunction, and urinary/bowel control may add to low self-worth

fear of secondary injury: always a possiblity, but more so when there is loss of sensation, pain, and temperature appreciation for hot and cold

About themselves. People with disabilities often feel fear (I can't take care of myself, no one will want to take care of me), self-doubt, worthlessness, failure (I can't stand tall, do my work, take care of my family, compete), self-hate, rage at self, others, the gods. Their wishes include that that there will be more accessbility everywhere, to buildings, on public transportation, in restaurants and restrooms, to the height of water fountains and work desks, in the streets with curb cuts, in stores with wider aisles.

About you. People with disabilities feel discomfort when the able-bodied are uncomfortable with them. They feel forebearance (another idiot!), envy (I wish I were healthy, able-bodied, on my feet, both of them), and anger. They wish you would learn to respect them as individuals, find out about their abilities, inform yourself about disabilities, and react intelligently instead of ignorently and emotionally. A disability is an inconvenient fact, not a character description; a part of life, not a way of life.

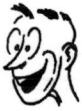 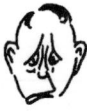 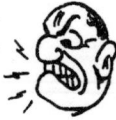 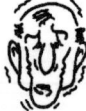 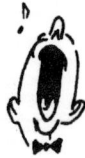

HAPPY   SAD   ANGRY   NERVOUS   SINGING

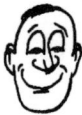 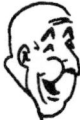 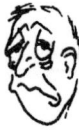 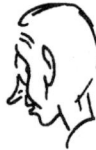 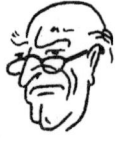

POLITE   OOPS!   TIRED   SHY   SERIOUS

If you can't speak your feelings, you can point to them.

YOUR FEELINGS

About people with disabilities, your feelings will probably begin with feeling nervous, and uncomfortable.

Common feelings are:

I don't know why, but I'm afraid

I don't know what to do

I don't know what to say

I don't know where to look

I don't know how to act

I want to help

I don't know if my help is wanted

I don't want to make a mistake

I don't want to give offense

I don't know if your mind is affected as well as your
body and if it is, how to communicate

But I'm interested in, and curious about, the condition:
what's wrong? how do you live like that? what
kind of life can you have?

And — had I better suppress or subdue my own
enthusiasms, my own vitality around you?

Deeper feelings may include:

Fear: it could happen to me

Anxiety over contagion: I could get it

Relief: thankfulness it isn't me

Superiority: someone I can feel better than

Inferiority: their cross to bear is greater than mine

Desire to avoid: I don't want to feel what I'm feeling and
don't know what to do about it

Desire to help: I have to do something

Identification: well, really, we're all human beings

Compassion: a true sorrow and affection

All of these feelings are less acute if someone you see or
meet in a wheelchair or on crutches, or who is using a prosthesis
such as a mechanical arm or hand, foot, or leg, appears other-
wise in control. If someone is spastic with cerebral palsey, or
appears to have mental retardation, or seems in any other way
not in control, the feelings are more acute. This may be particularly true also if there is deformity of limbs, or disfigurement as in

burn disabilities.

As someone close to the disabled, you may experience what is called caregiver syndrome: anger (at god, the doctors, the universe that it had to happen to your loved one and you); grief (at the loss of your old relationship and companionship, perhaps of someone who had been taking care of you); fear (of degeneration and death, of not being able to cope); exhaustion (from doing too much of the physical and psychological work, from too much responsibility, from loneliness).

Physical disability isn't necessarily the real disability in our lives. It can be a challenge to ingenuity, to spiritual strength, and a way to serve and inspire.

Real disability is deliberate cruelty, callous indifference, and the stupor of unexamined lives.

3

MANNERS THAT MATTER

Disability can overwhelm us with feelings: those who have the disability as well as those near them.

Unfortunately, most people, whether they have a physical disability or not, don't know how to share their feelings directly. We use comforting phrases, instead of truly listening. We act out by attack and withdrawal instead of trying honesty. And instead of understanding, we pass judgment. Our manners, on both sides, can be pretty awful.

Saying what you feel, need, perceive is necessary to communication, and it is based on self-awareness. Manners are based on the skill of stating these feelings, needs, perceptions without blame or judgment, and **only when and to whom it is appropriate.**

YOUR MANNERS

Don't stare.

Looking is fine. We all look at each other. But someone with a visible disability, a burn or birth deformity, is no more on display than any other person.

Don't avoid.

No one likes to be ignored.

Don't display discomfort.

Remind yourself there is a person there, not just a disability. No one wants to feel like a belled leper. Even if you are uncomfortable, control your overreactions.

Don't invade.

"Hi, what's the matter with you?" is as unpardonable an intrusion as any other personal question. If and when it is appropriate, information may be volunteered, even requested delicately. Be sensitive to when it is time to back off.

Don't be effusive or emotional.

Don't rain your own feelings all over other people's disabilities. They probably don't feel sorry for themselves.

Ask before offering help.

The urge is natural. Trespassing is not.

Don't make people with disabilities different.

As Kathy Buckley, the standup comedien who happens to be deaf as well as very funny, always says, "Don't pass any judgment you wouldn't want passed on yourself. Treat us, and think of us, like anyone else."

THEIR MANNERS

Rudeness is not exclusive to the able-bodied. People with disabilities can be equally out of sorts. Disability does not confer sainthood. If the able-bodied stare or behave offensively, it should come as no surprise if someone with a disability is not amused.

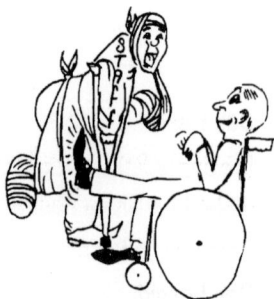

A spasm is not an excuse for battering

Kindness and graciousness.

Some people with disabilities may have been cutting up their own salads or crossing streets or going to the bathroom on their own for years. But the next disabled person may have a genuine need, and it isn't necessary to permanently thwart a possibly genuine source of help for other handicapped souls. Remember, when the uninformed able-bodied are awkward, it is because they are stupified by their fear that what's the matter with the disabled could happen to them. It's better to be gracious and kind.

SHARING INFORMATION

If you are a friend to or a person who takes care of someone with a disability, you will rapidly become an expert in how to understand and attend to what problems are involved.

Learn to share experiences, strength, and information whenever and wherever the opportunity presents itself.

You can help the disabled to campaign for accessibility to public buildings, their rights to employment, against prejudice, ignorance, and the massive indifference that can be the greatest obstacle of all.

You can encourage and help the disabled to act as role models, so that everyone can learn a disability may not be the end of anything at all.

People with handicaps often feel separated from the rest of the world. Rehabilitation teaches those with an injury or illness or genetic defect to make ordinary lives for themselves. It is up to those with disabilities to teach the world how possible this is.

A boy I knew with a facial burn deformity wore a mask. Partly, this was so the sun would not blister his face while he was skiing. Partly, it was from consideration and purpose.

"It's so I don't frighten other people. I have a lot to say, a lot to share, and a lot of life to live."

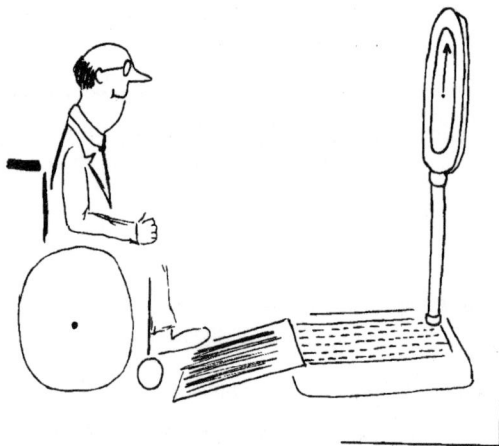

4
SEEKING DIAGNOSES

Medical school and the miracles of modern medical technology have taught physicians to respect science. They are trained to measure data, and to draw conclusions based on scientific observation about medical issues and medical treatment.

What the medical doctor often ignores are the valuable life experiences, observations, and feelings of clients about themselves and their own conditions. This often has disastrous results on correct diagnoses and treatment, the proper fitting and functioning of wheelchairs and prosthetics, as well as the prescription of medications, and the course of appropriate rehabilitation.

There is the story of a famous artist Chuck Close, for instance, who was in rehabilitation at an equally famous hospital after being paralyzed from the neck down. When partial use of his forearms returned, he was being taught by an OT to do his laundry. Until he exploded that he had never done or ever planned on doing his own laundry, no one had bothered to ask.

RELATING TO DOCTORS

There are things all of us need to know about consultations with doctors. But friends of the disabled need to be doubly aware because of the greater complications involved. This is particularly true for primary caregivers.

• You can be very useful and helpful as a friend or caregiver if you accompany your disabled friend or relative to the doctor.

• Choose physicians who listen, who question their clients' experience of themselves, their physical symptoms, their psychological states.

• Be responsible for effective communication about problems and needs. Doctors may be sensitive, but they do not mind-read.

answer exactly the questions the doctor asks: doctors know what they want to know

don't overload the doctor with extraneous complaints

be prepared with your information and your questions

be clear in your information and as precise and accurate as possible about your symptoms

insist you understand clearly what the doctor says to you: you'll be facing the "what did the doctor say" question from loved ones later on

• Be ample with your information within the confines of your appointment.

Try to be alert to a doctor's prejudices concerning gender, intellect, or race. A doctor, for instance, might hear complaints differently from a man or a woman, the rich or the poor, one race or religion or ethnic background over another, the young or the old, the fat or the thin, the whole or the infirm (and since prejudices are strange, preferences might surprise you!).

Some doctors, like some parents, measure their success by your improvement. Be careful not to deny your pain and take it home with you yet again in order to prove you are a *good* client and win your doctor's approval.

But it is also true that clients have peculiarities above and beyond their particular conditions. Be as aware of your own conditioning and character defects as you expect your doctors to be.

In short:

1. Be clear about your symptoms
2. Be clear about what you think you need from the doctor
3. Press for what you need
4. Don't settle for a doctor you don't like, don't trust, don't feel you can talk to and be heard by, if you can possibly help it.
5. Cooperate: the doctor or therapist can't do it all
6. Get a second opinion. Doctors are not all equal.

Clients need more than a wheelchair and medication, a spare leg or an iron lung, a course of physical and occupational rehabilitation. Clients need to receive affectionate guidance and encouragement — and need to give it. A good doctor-patient relationship may be based on the doctor's medical knowledge and your need of that knowledge, but the outcome is based on your common humanity, your trust, and your affection for one another.

Coping with the health-care system is complex enough to imperial your sanity. To be passed from one doctor to another, one facility or rehabilitation center to another, the navigation through a sea of paper work, from doctor to insurance company, from hospital to outpatient care, the testing and fitting of adaptive equipment, the constant need for medical attention, special supplies, exercise and diet supervision, often psychotherapy as well as physical therapy — it's a life that depends on the very sanity it threatens.

That makes it all the more reason to be persistent, to find the doctor or doctors, the physical therapists, the psychotherapists, the treatment centers, the rehabilitation experts, the adaptive equipment technologists, in whatever fields of work or interest are needed, with the breath of kindness in them, whose diagnoses and advice you can trust and respect. Get referrals and recommendations, interview when possible, quit and move on if necessary.

Just don't give up.

CHOOSING DOCTORS AND FACILITIES

If the disability was genetic or caused by the birth process, chances are it was tracked from the beginning by the obstetrician, health-care system, social workers, at the hospital of birth.

If the disability was acquired later on or only presented itself later on, and you need to choose a physician, call the following for recommendations:

- National associations serving your injury or illness
- Nearest hospital or good university medical school
- Friends, family doctor, minister, rabbi, priest, and others you trust for referrals

5

LIVING WITH A PHYSICAL DISABILITY:
A DAY IN A WHEELCHAIR
True Life Stories

Life is tough enough. It can be made nearly impossible for someone in a wheelchair, on quad forearm crutches, canes, or walkers, with braces or artificial limbs. Many people with prosthetic devices and adaptive equipment are unable to go up or down five flights of stairs, use a bathroom with no handrails or too tiny to turn in or transfer from a chair, enter doorways too narrow for wheelchairs to enter rooms or elevators, or navigate tight aisles in stores, on trains, in movie theaters.

The original trauma can often be managed by relying on an indomitable spirit, or on the support of friends and family.

It's the deadening reality of the kind of slow, day-after-day struggle with absent, weakened, paralyzed, or spastic limbs, the chronic fatigue or pain, the need for a respirator to breathe that drags at the spirit.

It's what happens when the body suffers from lack of use and muscles become thin and weak, leg bones become porous and break easily, circulation is poor, the heart and lungs are affected, and internal organs like the kidneys and bladder are dysfunctional and easily infected.

It's the constant extra needs for body maintenance, like electronic muscle stimulation that can help strengthen muscle tissue and increase bone density.

It's the need for catheters and medication and suppositories, pads and pampers, the prayer to win the race for the bathroom.

High-tech science has built lovely limbs for amputee models, legs for marathon runners, hands for artists, new "bones" for the old, computers so the blind can read Braille printouts, and aids for the deaf to hear. There's everything to experiment with, from the Seattle Foot, the OKC Running Leg, the Sabolich Socket, high tech knees, the Delrin plastic foot arch, and the energy-storing Quantum Foot, to Steeper Myoelectric Hands, the Boston Arm, or the Utah Arm. There's the Zap Mobile, the sports wheel-chairs, walking harnesses with FNS controls.

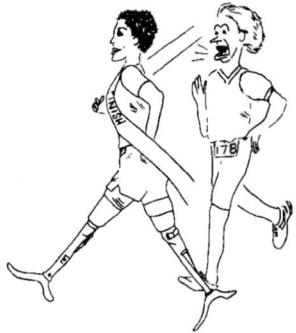

Sabolich Foot

But no matter how exciting and sophisticated our adaptive equipment grows, how clever our motion and environmental aids become, how customized our equipment for jobs, cars, and tools, daily life can still be a grind.

JOHN CALLAHAN — cartoonist, author of
Don't Worry, He Won't Get Far On Foot

Quadriplegic, alcoholic, former bum with an uproarious,

black sense of humor, Callahan describes in his book everything from how a quadriplegic has sex to the horror show of the welfare system. His description of his first days of trying independent living after rehab with his first live-in attendant is a nightmare.

It took an attendant three hours to get him up, attend to catheter and bowel program, wash, dress, get him into corset, support stockings, wrist braces, and with Callahan hanging onto the trapeze above his hospital bed, out of the bed and into his wheelchair.

MARY VERDI-FLETCHER — dancer, founder of *Dancing Wheels*

At twelve, after ten operations related to her spina bifida, a spinal disability from birth, Mary almost died of acute decubitus — bedsores. Confined to a wheelchair for life, she began to go out dancing with a friend, competed with her partner on a national TV show as the first able-bodied/disabled dance team, founded Dancing Wheels, became involved with the Cleveland Ballet, and conducts a dance workshop for young children.

CHUCK CLOSE — artist

Quadriplegic from collapsed spinal artery, Close is grateful to paint again from a partial return of his muscles, plus the use of an orthotic device with Velcro so he can use a brush, and a forklift truck to get to the tops of his paintings.

He uses quad-crutches as well as a wheelchair. His painting life, he says, because he can get help, equipment, and various devices made, is the most normal part of his life. But he can't roughhouse with his young daughter, or be the companion he once was to his wife. It hurts physically to sit all day, to have bladder infections. It hurts psychologically to go to the theater, and look down to see he has a lap full of urine, or to get handicapped tickets for Carnegie Hall and find the seat is down ten steps and five places in. Where he lives and works in New York, there are few curb cuts, and everything is up two or three steps. There is nearly no handicapped parking.

Most important to him of all is, he says, "I want to have my paintings judged with the best paintings, not just people who are handicapped. I want to be seen just as an artist."

TONY MELENDEZ — guitarist

His mother took the drug thalidomide as a sedative during her pregnancy. Melendez was born without arms. In the handicapped schools, everyone had something different wrong with them — children were in wheelchairs, on crutches, blind. He needed the attention that teachers in a public school wouldn't know how to give. Teachers simply put the pencil in between his toes. Whatever he could get hold of with his feet, he tried. He writes, dresses, cooks, drives a car (the wheel is on the floor next to the gas and brake).

Children ask him, "Where are your arms?" He says, "Got none." They are curious, they want to know. "Why not?" they say.

Some people are bothered by his presence. He isn't bothered by them. What slows him down is that things aren't where he needs them to be, like doorknobs. He would rather they were

29

at the bottom of the doors. No matter what is taken away from you, Melendez says, something else will take over.   Just work. Don't give up.   On the one hand, he can't manage a paper plate. On the other, he sang for the pope.

SENIORS WITH DISABILITIES

We are blessed, in the West, with the means and the technology to prolong life. An even greater blessing might be an improvement in the manners and attitudes that make a longer life worth living.

HELEN GRANT — teacher, senior citizen

Helen Grant is a friend in her late eighties. Both of her legs have been amputated, one above and one below the knee, due to complications from diabetes.

She is an independent woman by temperament. She drives a car with hand controls, does her own marketing and errands. Her life had been spent as a teacher, and she continues to give lectures and take part in community life as well as to travel. She is perfectly mobile in her wheelchair. What she resents most, when she goes where she is not known, is that her credibility, intelligence, and competence are often questioned by people who make what she calls idiotic assumptions "that my mind was amputated along with my legs."

CHILDREN WITH DISABILITIES

There are children who have lived with their disabilities since they were born. There are children who are victims of terrible accidents and diseases. Several million of them have survived triumphantly their surgeries and physical therapy, institutionalization, medications, pain, terror, loneliness, being stared at, ignored, infantilized. Their suffering, and that of their friends and families, has only been exceeded by their courage and endurance.

The names have been changed.

JANE: Jane's parents were killed in an automobile accident in which she too was involved. After a year of surgeries and rehabilitation, she came home to her brothers and older sister, strapped into a wheelchair. A spinal column injury damaged nerves, and although she can use a standing board with an attached desktop in school so her muscles don't tighten up too much and a walker around the house, both are too tiring to use for long. She swims. She plays tennis. When she gets mad at people, she runs over their feet with her wheelchair.

What she hates is that her older sister has to come to school to catheterize her in the school bathroom.

HOLLY: Holly had a birth defect that left her with one normal leg, and one leg that required amputation. She wears an artificial leg on her stump. She wears a liner, a plastic suction socket held in a

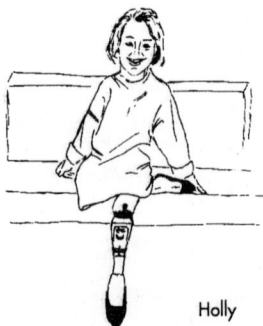

Holly

graphite frame with a hydraulic knee and a Flex-Foot. She does not cover her Flex-Foot when she competes: it unsettles her opponents. She set world records in races for the physically challenged, and prefers international competitions in other countries because she thinks other cultures are less ignorant about people with disabilities.

BOBBY: Bobby has dwarfism, one of 150 kinds of this condition. His dwarfism is achondroplastic like 80% of dwarfs. This means his head is normal size, but his arms and legs are shortened, he has problems with bones and circulation, respiratory problems, troubles with his hands, and other medical problems that often require operations. He spends a lot of time in his wheelchair. But even when he's not in his wheelchair, everything in a world built for tall people is a problem from legs reaching the floor from a chair, to hands reaching a sink tap from the floor. Stools and special pulls all over the house help him manage. Clothes that never fit can be made. But people treating him like a baby because he's small, or like a dimwit because they think "small body, small brain," makes him mad.

GRAHAM: Graham was born with a genetic disability that results in having no arms or legs. His hands come from his shoulders. He has stumps for legs because the doctors thought he might be able to use

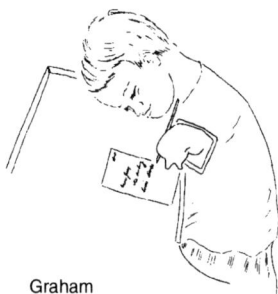

Graham

32

artificial legs if they amputated the flippers he was born with. He can eat, brush his teeth, and writes with his fingers, as well as work at his computer. His mother uses adaptive equipment so he can pour his own milk, and get things for himself around the house. He has prosthetic legs built like short boots to wear over his stumps to school, but they're tiring to wear and cause rashes when they rub. At home, he walks on his stumps. He uses an electric wheelchair most of the time.

Graham goes to a school for kids with disabilities where everything is adapted for people in wheelchairs and where along with the regular schoolwork, he does occupational and physical therapy. He needs help getting into his wheelchair and into his legs. When he's late, he carries his legs wherever he's going and gets help putting them on at the other end. Graham wishes people would just treat him like any other human being.

A NOTE ABOUT FRIENDS, LOVERS, SPOUSES, FAMILIES

All of this is hard on families and friends, too. It isn't always easy to remember to treat disabled loved ones for their essential selves and to treat the disability as secondary. Healthy caretakers have to put out ten times the wattage if a spouse has MS, or a healthy sibling gets ten times less attention than a handicapped brother or sister. Death, genetic possibilities for future generations of children, infections, bills, caretaker exhaustion and loneliness are haunting spectres.

The expenses are enormous, in addition to funding, and often seriously deplete a family's resources. To say nothing of the heartache you feel when yet another ignoramus hurts feelings, slams doors, fails to provide courtesies if not necessities to your loved one.

But living in pain or partial immobility in our speeded-up and usually unaccommodating world affects those with the disabilities the most.

I have a friend, paralyzed ,who uses a wheelchair, who says the panic never leaves; he never gets used to the lack of sensation or his physical near-helplessness: as if, he says, he had been buried alive.

But Richard Fucci, who sustained a spinal cord injury in 1977, who has been actively involved in issues concerning persons with disabilities ever since, who has served as president of The National Spinal Cord Injury Association and helped to found the Sail Connecticut Access Program to provide sailing opportunities for people with disabilities, Richard Fucci says, "In some situations, my lack of mobility can lead to near-panic and a lack of accessibility, like a hotel reservation that turns out to be on the fourteenth floor (you know, the first thing they do if there is a fire is shut the elevators off) well, then, naturally panic sets in. But normally, my life doesn't have any more anxious moments than anyone else's."

When I mention that one of life's most extraordinary mysteries is the capacity many people have to find a redemptive meaning to suffering and adapt, even to triumph over pain, he adds, "There's nothing redemptive about being a quad."

6

RESOURCES: ADAPTIVE AND MOBILITY AIDS; BIONIC PARTS;
REHABILITATION; DIET AND EXERCISE; RETRAINING; NEW
TRAINING; THE WORKPLACE AND ADA; FUNDS

The human body is a living machine. It is run by an extraordinary computer we call the brain, along a network of nerves. The body machine, directed by the brain, pumps life-giving blood to all its parts, even grows new tissues to replace and repair its own structures, skin, muscles, bones.

The body machine also breaks down. Defect, disease, accidental injury, burns, age, overuse and overloading — anything can break it, or cause a systems failure.

The brain then invents miracles: drugs to help the body fight pain and infection; physical, occupational, psychotherapeutic rehabilitation techniques to put the body back in the mainstream; exercises, electronic stimulation, and diets to strengthen and maintain it; and for what it can-

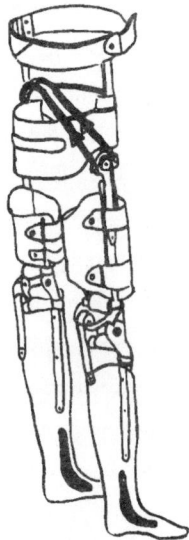

LSU High
Tech Leg Brace

not repair on its own, various devices for whatever disabilities the machine has incurred.

WHEELCHAIRS

They can be the most expensive of all orthopedic equipment. Know what you need, as it is almost impossible to get third-party payers, like insurance companies, to cover you a second time. Wheelchairs must fit the body's needs and through the bathroom door, adapt to the disability, to the workplace, to the van, to the environment, to favorite activities. A wheelchair that is too low to the ground, presses on the pelvic bone, or doesn't have the appropriate controls, is a torment.

The advice of a doctor, or a physical or occupational therapist, is mandatory. Information about a client's disability and needs, size and posture, are necessary. There is a great deal of difference between a simple transport chair and a permanent, functional chair; a chair for someone with paraplegia or quadriplegia. There are power chairs and scooters. There are chairs with breath controls. There are chairs with removable armrests for transfers, lightweight chairs with easily removable wheels for traveling. There are chairs with pressure gauges to cushion properly against bedsores, that answer all postural needs. There are chairs that answer various other specifications: questions of transportation, whether the client drives herself and needs to fold up her own chair, or requires a van-fitting chair; questions of varying disabilities.

If the chair does not fit properly, pressure sores, back and

36

head and neck pains result. Or there are mechanical and logistical difficulties; the seat can be so low the client cannot stand up, for instance. If it is an electronically controlled chair, the computer and its controls for severely disabled clients must be correctly positioned to adjust everything from room temperature to TV to telephone.

There are adaptive chairs for dancing, for sports, from monoskis to marathons. The possibilities, in today's medical technology, are remarkable.

ORTHOTICS

Some adaptive aids do not need to be fitted. But orthopedic aids such as walkers, canes, crutches, braces, splints, all positioning and ambulatory aids, do need to be fitted and supervised by a physical therapist. The manufacturers of off-the-shelf, one-size-fits-all orthotic devices in stores or catalogues, usually manage to fit no one exactly right. The results can range from uncomfortable blisters and infection to disastrous falls.

Equipment is available from medical-equipment stores, by mail from health-supply catalogs, or through a hospital physical-therapy unit. Again, check with your trained medical professional first.

Canes and crutches.

Standard cane — lightweight aluminum or heavier, natural woods, canes come in all shapes and sizes

Quad canes — simple form with handle offset with foam grip; three- and four-pointed canes for balance

Quad forearm crutch — comes with an adjustable fitting that

fastens over the length of the forearm

Walkers.

Usually aluminum, walkers are wheeled, folding, or rigid. They are even more secure balancing aids than canes and crutches.

Splints and braces.

These are now made of lightweight plastic and Velcro for legs, arms, hands, feet, head, and neck.

Adaptive equipment.

Catalogues are full of adaptive devices to assist people sitting in wheelchairs, with balance problems, reaching problems. Devices range from dressing aids to bathroom, kitchen, bed, worktable devices, transfer boards, adapted furniture, sports and exercise equipment, toys and learning aids, games, children's and adult's standers, walkers, positioning equipment.

BIONIC PARTS

The designs for artificial limbs for amputees are revolutionary. New custom limbs can be mechanically activated or electrically stimulated. From cosmetically impeccable, lifelike arms,

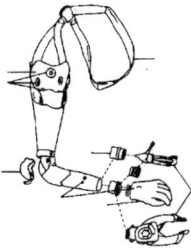

Utah arm

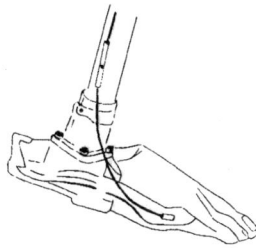

Quantum Foot

hands, legs, and feet to computer waist packs, implanted electrodes, and Functional Neuromuscular Stimulation, modern technological research has enabled people with amputated or paralyzed limbs to stand, walk, climb again.

REHABILITATION

The word means to restore to a former state or capacity, to restore to a condition of health, or useful and constructive activity.

Doctors, physical therapists, occupational therapists, psychotherapists, and a battery of specialists in related fields all conspire to help people with disabilities live as normal and independent a life as possible, in the mainstream if possible, as soon as possible.

Rehabilitation centers may be part of hospital complexes, or separate centers, or research centers. They may be oriented toward one or another disability or specific rehabilitation field.

Gaylord, in Wallingford, Connecticut, is an excellent example of a not-for-profit Rehabilitation Hospital, affiliated with Yale University School of Medicine. It is devoted to treating people who have been disabled by illness or injury, and who can benefit from comprehensive rehabilitation. There are inpatient and outpatient services that include rehabilitation for:

Traumatic Brain Injury	Industrial Rehabilitation
Spinal Cord Injury	Chemical Dependency
Stroke and Pulmonary	General Rehabilitation

Outpatient services include:

- ADA Consultation
- Gaylord Regional Prosthetics/Orthotics Center
- Hand Rehabilitation
- Multiple Sclerosis Clinic
- Occupational Therapy
- Pain Management Rehabilitation
- Physiatry
- Physical Therapy
- Post-Polio Assessment
- Return to Work Services
- Sexuality/Infertility Counseling
- Social Work
- Sports Medicine Physical Therapy
- Transitional Living
- Vocational Services
- Wheelchair Services
    And much more....

DIET AND EXERCISE

Just as the occupational therapist's continued suggestions for safety and modifications are necessary for comfort in the daily activities of living, proper diet and exercise for people in wheelchairs are necessary for health. Physical inactivity makes the body prone to pressure sores, stiffness, poor circulation, respiratory problems, and apathy.

Many people with physical disabilities today are turning off the television set and choosing the fun and challenge of active lives in physical recreation, even hard-driving national and international competition. One Director of Rehabilitation, himself disabled, says, "I reject the medical model of illness and go for it. It's our responsibility to help people perceive us the way we want to be perceived. Let's focus on our abilities, not our disabilities, and get out there."

S.A.R.A.H., the Shoreline Association for the Retarded and Handicapped, along with its group homes, employment services, and many other rehabilitation programs; has a daily community enrichment program for those in need of total care. It includes physical and occupational therapy, and also the going out into the community, its shops and restaurants, banks and hairdressers, places of employment, concerts and movies and sports events, so that everybody sees, is seen by, and included in the common life of the whole.

RETRAINING; NEW TRAINING; THE WORKPLACE AND ADA
(AMERICANS WITH DISABILITIES ACT)

Robert Blake, the actor, said during a television program called *Taking Charge: People with Disabilities,*

"There is no such thing as a handicapped soul."

There are many Resource Centers for the Handicapped in Canada and the United States for retraining and new training of people with disabilities in old or new, vocational and occupational work.

There are two main problems:

1. Bosses do not realize it is cheaper to take back or take on a

41

trained disabled worker than to train a new person in the job. (The average cost of reasonable workplace accommodation according to ADA specifications for equal access is about $500 per person — a wider door, a lower water cooler.)

2. It is harder to change attitudes than the workplace. Many people continue to confuse a disability with illness, or to think people with disabilities are tragic victims.

Facts:

• there are nearly 50 million disabled people in the United States

• 76% of them are unemployed

• the cost of this to the nation is $200 billion (about the size of the defense budget)

• people with disabilities are just that, people who would rather be working and living in the mainstream than isolated and dependent on welfare

• the Americans with Disabilities Act prohibits discrimination in the workplace, but it can only open up doors, not minds — ADA describes and further prohibits the persistent discrimination experienced by people with disabilities:

　　　　1. in employment, housing, public accommodations, education, transportation, communication, recreation, health services, access to public services, even voting

　　　　2. outright, intentional exclusion, segregation or relegation to lesser programs, and architectural, transportation, and communication barriers

　　　　3. included in their description are people for whom

public prejudice may constitute a disability: those with HIV virus, people with facial disfigurement that is disabling only because of the attitudes and reactions of others

• opening minds needs to begin with early education, as in the Avon, CT school where children with disabilities are not separated out, where 10% of the children have special needs, are each given an aide, and take their places in class where their classmates learn early to include everyone in their community — educators are learning this prevents the group from developing the fears and prejudices that most people have toward the disabled

MYTHS PERSIST: **we can stop them and investigate the facts instead**
WE CAN ALSO REMEMBER: **we are all only temporarily able-bodied**

FUNDS

Disability, whether genetic or acquired, is usually very costly.

For funding, the best information will come from your local rehabilitation center or hospital, your doctor, and the appropriate national disability organization.

There is public assistance for persons with disabilities, medical assistance instead of insurance, whether you are orthopedically handicapped, other handicapped, multiple-handicapped, technology-dependent. There are sources for independent living with an attendant, group homes, rehabilitation centers, nursing homes, hospitals with inpatient and outpatient services. A list of some of these have been added at the end of the book.

43

7

FIX YOUR ATTITUDE AS WELL AS YOUR HOUSE
ADAPT!   ADAPT!   ADAPT!

Adaptive technology for people with disabilities is miraculous and available. Its amazing gifts range from respirators and replacement hearts, limbs, and other parts to a sensible pair of oak planks to turn your front steps into a wheelchair-accessible ramp through your front door.

It's our attitudes that need the help. Here are some positive things you can do.

1. Remember, while you are improving access, to improve inter-action. Curiosity is good: it is the antidote to closed-minded prejudice. Ask and answer questions. "Understand, however," says Richard Fucci, "that the disability may hold only a fraction of the interest of whoever has it and will certainly not be what he or she wants most to be remembered for or base a friendship on."

2. Offer assistance, but do not insist; do not help without permission, ask about choices, never presume on another person's body needs, and if you are not certain what is needed, ask for an explanation.

3. Be aware of limitations, but never assume someone with a disability can or cannot do something. Do not prohibit someone from taking risks because you are nervous about the disability. There is never failure — only attempts that don't work and work

that can be started all over again.

4. Remember the power of words: concentrate on remembering we are all people first; our attributes are secondary. Someone uses a wheelchair (not, is wheelchair-bound), someone has a disability (not, is disabled). Avoid condescending euphemisms (physically challenged), as well as words that connote disease or illness (patients).

5. Avoid shouting at someone in a wheelchair as if she were also deaf or incompetent, referring to someone in a wheelchair in his presence as if he were a child, or talking over her head as if to pretend she were standing up like everyone else in the room. Acknowledge people in a wheelchair with the same accommodation and courtesy you would give anyone else.

(Remember: they are driving a weapon that, when handled properly, can run you over, break your kneecaps, and put you where they're sitting now.)

6. Try not to segregate people with disabilities. They want to get on with their lives just like everyone else according to their interests, abilities, needs, and desires.

7. Don't spend every waking moment thinking of nothing but their disabilities. They don't.

PEOPLE WITH DISABILITIES SURVIVE THE SAME WAY EVERY-
ONE ELSE DOES, BY HAVING A PATHOLOGICAL OPTIMISM,
BY REFUSING TO DIE, TO GIVE IN, TO GIVE UP.

FOR ALL OF US, CREATING ONE'S OWN LIFE IS A VOYAGE
INTO THE UNKNOWN.

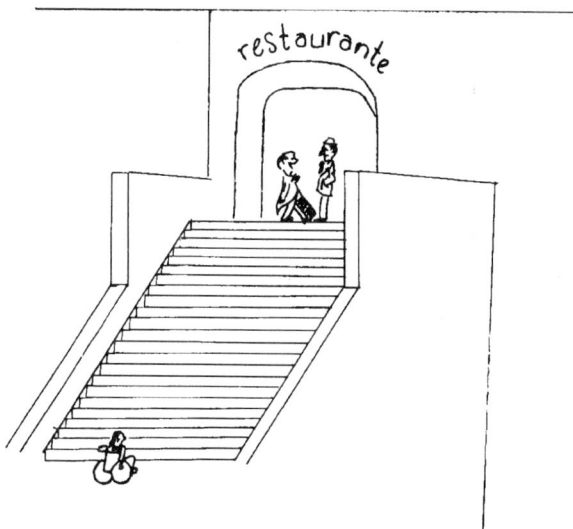

We don't need a ramp because the handicapped don't come here anyway.

SOURCES FOR HELP

It is important to join disability, illness, injury, birth defect associations. This helps to support research and services. The association can provide lists of support groups, of literature, books, pamphlets, magazines, medical journal articles, as well as local organizations and specialized organizations such as for sports, or the arts, for each disability.

Remember, the local rehabilitation facilities in your area offer programs from pain management to sex to recreational opportunities, in addition to the obvious treatment and adaptive technology.

Disability organizations

Adaptive Environments Center, 374 Congress Street, Suite 301, Boston, MA 02210. (617) 695-1225.

American Amputee Foundation, P.O. Box 55218, Hillcrest Station, Little Rock, AR 72225. (501) 666-2523, (800) 553-4483.

Association of Birth Defect Children, Orlando Executive Park, Suite 270, 5400 Diplomat Circle, Orlando, FL 32810. (407) 629-1466.

Barrier Free Environments, In., P.O. Box 30634, U.S. Highway 70, West Water Garden, Raleigh, NC 27622. (919) 782-7823.

Clearinghouse on the Handicapped, Office of Special Education and Rehabilitative Services, Room 3132, Switzer Building, Washington, DC 20202. (202) 732-1245.

Little People of America, P.O. Box 9897, Washington, DC 20016. (301) 589-0730.

National Chronic Pain Outreach Association, 7979 Old Georgetown Road, Suite 100, Bethesda, MD 20814. (301) 652-4948.

National Council on Independent Living, Troy Atrium, 4th Street and Broadway, Troy, NY 12180. (518) 274-1979.

National Organization on Disability, 910 16th Street, N.W., Washington, DC 20006. (800) 248-ABLE, (202) 5960.

National Rehabilitation Information Center, 8455 Colesville Road, #935, Silver Spring, MD 22091. (800) 34-NARIC.

National Spinal Cord Injury Association, 600 West Cummings Park, Suite 2000, Woodburn, MA 01801. (800) 962-9629.

Rehabilitation International, The International Society for Rehabilitation of the Disabled, 25 East 21st Street, New York, NY 10010. (212) 420-1500.

Government agencies:

National Council on Disability, 800 Independence Avenue, S.W., Suite 814, Washington, DC 20591. (202) 267-3235.

National Information Center for Children and Youth with Disabilities, P.O. 1492, Washington, DC 20013. (703) 893-6061. (800) 999-5599.

Rehabilitation Services Administration, U.S. Department of Education, 330 C Street, S.W. Washington, DC 20001. (202) 732-1282.

There are:

Arts and disability organizations:
Very Special Arts, an educational affiliate of the John F. Kennedy Center for the Performing Arts, (800) 933-8721.

Athletic organizations:
International, national, and local sports associations serve each disability, with teaching clinics, and competitive events for each disability, for those who have amputations, who have cerebral palsy, who have spinal-cord injuries, who have dwarfism, who have multiple sclerosis, muscular dystrophy, and others. All of them have junior divisions.

These are a few of the national disabled sports organizations:

National Handicapped Sports (for amputees in summer sports, and all groups in winter sports), 4405 East-West Highway, Suite 603, Bethesda, MD 20814. (301) 652-7505.

National Wheelchair Athletic Association, 3617 Betty Drive, Suite S, Colorado Springs, CO 80907. (719) 597-8330.

The above listing is partial and general. There are organizations for every disability. Check with your local hospital, library, or use the above list to begin your inquiry for more information.

For adaptive devices and equipment, prostheses information, there are many catalogues and magazines such as *Ability*, with a Yellow Pages listing of national and regional support centers.

You can write or call **Able Data** (Newington Children's Hospital), 181 E. Cedar Street, Newington, CT 06111. (800) 344-5405, (203) 667-5405. Funded by the National Institute on Disability and Rehabilitation Research, AbleData maintains a database with over 15,000 listings of adaptive devices for all disabilities.

You can write or call ADA Consulting-Compliance Design Co., 2244 West Coast HWY #200 Newport Beach, CA 92663. (714) 646-3756. CDC is a consulting firm which offers ADA compliance surveys and implementation plans to make businesses public and commercial facilities, local and state facilities accessible and in compliance with state and ADA requirements.

New Mobility is a magazine that addresses a broad range of issues for people with mobility impairments.

Resources for adaptive equipment:
Consumer Care Products, Sheboygan Falls, WI 53085. (414) 467-2393. Wheelchairs, bicycles, positioning devices, OT and PT supplies.

Flaghouse Special Populations Catalog, 150 North MacQueen Parkway, Mt. Vernon, NY 10550. (914) 329-6000. Products for body movements, self-sufficiency, learning toys and games.

Two extensive medical mail-order equipment catalogues:
Abbey Medical, 17390 Brookhurst St., #200, Fountain Valley, CA 92708.

Fred Sammons, P.O. Box 32, Brookfield, IL 60513.

Do not forget to consult your doctor, your physiatrist, your community-assistance organizations, and medical health-care professionals.

SELECTED REFERENCE BIBLIOGRAPHY

Callahan, John, *Don't Worry, He Won't Get Far On Foot,* New York, Vintage Books-Random House, 1990.

Carroll, David L. , and Jon Dudley Dorman, M.D., *Living Well with MS*, New York, HarperCollins, 1993.

Connaughton, Shane, and Jim Sheridan, *My Left Foot,* London, Boston, Faber and Faber, 1989.

Donohue, Paul J., Ph.D., and Mary E. Siegel, Ph.D., *Sick and Tired of Feeling Sick and Tired,* New York, W.W. Norton & Co., 1992.

Kettlekamp, Larry, *High Tech for the Handicapped,* Hillside, N.J., Enslow Publishers, Inc., 1991.

Krementz, Jill, *How It Feels to Live with a Physical Handicap,* New York, Simon & Schuster, 1992.

Rosenberg, Michael S., Ph.D., and Irene Edmond-Rosenberg, M.P.A., *The Special Education Sourcebook, A Teacher's Guide to Programs, Materials, and Information Sources*, Woodbine House, 1994.

Smith, Jean Kennedy (Founder of Very Special Arts), and George Plimpton, *Chronicles of Courage*, New York, Random House, 1993.

Tierney, Lawrence M., Jr., M.D., Stephen J. McPhee, M.D., and Maxine A. Papadakis, M.D., *Current Medical Diagnosis & Treatment*, Norwalk, CT, Appleton & Lange, 1995.

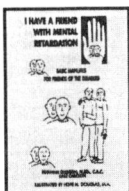

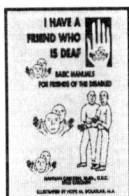

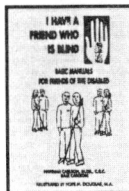

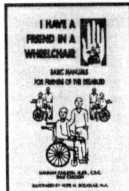

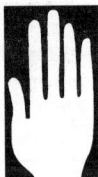

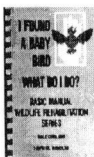

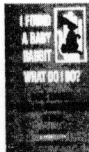

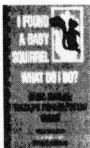

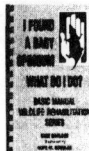

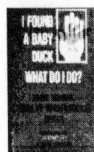

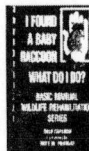